RESULTS MANUAL

The "How To" Manual For You To Take Results From Life!

By: Bertrand Ngampa

Who Is The Results Manual For?

I see you right now reading this book. But hold on, let me tell you something.

If you are looking how to get rich this is not the book, but you will learn more about your money from this book.

 If you are looking for the next fad diet this is not the book, but you will learn more about your food from this book.

If you are looking for God this not the book, but you will grow closer to God thru this book.

This book is your personal manual to help you maximize your results in each of your life pillars to help you reach your next level. (P.S life pillars are your mind, body, soul, and money)

Let me ask you..

Do you ever ask yourself, "is this all I can get out of my life?"

Do you go to your job day in and day out and wonder is this really my life?

Do you look in the mirror and are not pleased with what you see?

Have you built your mindset, properly planned your goals, created your action plans, and what about your personal affirmations?

Have you looked deeply and questioned your primary foods?

Have you started taking control of your money?

Do you know your money in and out?

Have you started to label money as the root of evil?

When is the last time you connected your mind, body, and soul?

Do you know and believe you are meant for more than where you are right now in life, but need the blueprint to access that more?

This Manual Is For You.

Don't be an information gatherer, but be a prolific action taker.

-Ryan Stewman

Results Be, On You!

About The Author

My name is Bertrand Harmen Ngampa. Known as Coach B, but please call me B.

I am not your standard think positive all the time and always happy coach.

My clients would tell you I am honest, edgy, and I expect them to win and get massive results. I carry their businesses, their visions, their whys, their families, their business goals, and personal goals as if they were my own.

I am different and just by you reading this manual you are now different too.

Growing up I was told I had to work harder and I was born to be different. I always fitted out instead of fitting in.

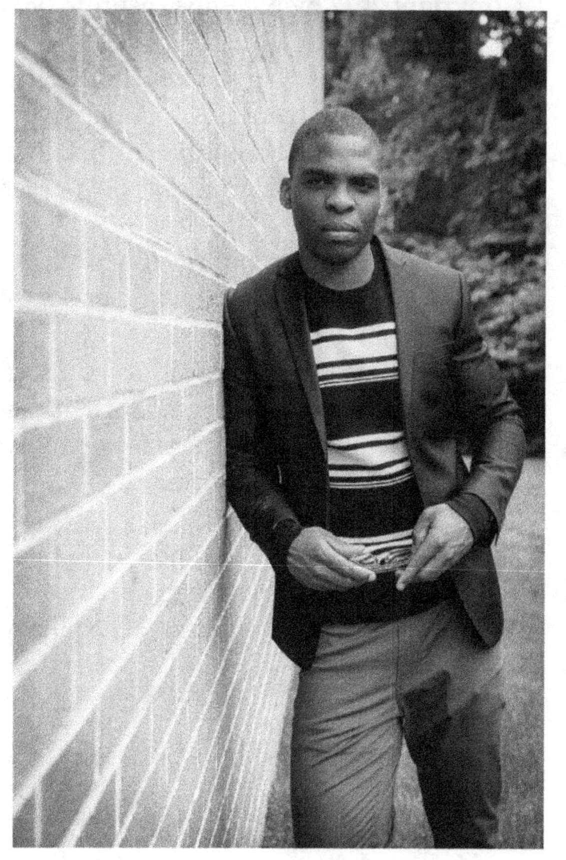

Before welcoming you to my world. My way of thinking, way of being, way of living and failing.

This book is your personal manual of how to achieve results in your life.

This book is short, but it will challenge you at all levels within your own life. This book will not give you any results. You must go out there and TAKE your results from life with the tools from this Manual!

I am a Man of God, an American Soldier, and now I am your Results Coach.

P.S My book cover looks good because April Rain James From Peridot Imagery. She does breathing take work for me and my clients.

 Http://www.peridotimagery.com

Book Cover: Peridot Imagery - April Rain James

RESULTS MANUAL OUTLINE

Foreword

Coach B and his Results Manual, B-FIT, is a clear pathway for helping you with your personal successes. He provides you with comprehensive and yet concise strategies of empowerment for the mind, soul and body. His infectious personality is heavily drenched within the composition of the book whereby it makes you feel as if you can hear him in your head and heart as you progress towards greater personal feats of victory for a better you, environment and economical freedom. Already half of my congregation has taken the course and they are seeing immediate benefits from his manual and presence within their lives. I encourage you to purchase this book. You will not regret this investment in his ministry and life. But also, you will tangibly see how the investment straightaway manifests even for your own life. That's only if you apprehend this book! I'm glad I did! It has elevated my thinking and healthy consciousness of living. And I'm certain this book has the necessities for the next phases of your life. For it has God's plan amongst it! And it provides a prophetic prelude to a greater realm of earthly and practical living. You won't regret connecting and learning from Coach B! He is a voice that has the influence necessary to take you to your next level of health, wholeness and a better fit tailor-made and intricately designed to properly define a better you!

Bishop-Elect Sherman D. Farmer

Presiding Prelate of New Gibeah Ministries for Christ Churches

Senior Pastor and Founder of the Cathedral on the Hill

Capital Heights, Maryland

The Bertrand Ngampa Short Story

Before you read this book and enter my world. I want to introduce myself to you. My name is Bertrand Harmen Ngampa. I am an American Soldier, Army Paratrooper "Airborne", Published Author, Result Coach, Man of God but most of all I am a human just like you. I have been at the top of the world and I have been at the bottom still climbing out. This book is my manual to you when you want to get results in your life. I have used theses methods time and time again in my own personal life.

Let's switch gear so I can tell you a little more about me, I was born in 1992 and lived in many different states and even overseas in Africa for a short brief time.

Growing up in the 90's was simple for me. I played with my brother Serge outside every day, did my homework, and went to church on Sunday. As I got older I realized we didn't have all the money in the world, because kids at school would tease me for not wearing the latest trendy shoes, having "Walmart clothes", and being black. (P.S black kids HATED me growing up, but white kids loved me.)

Growing up a little black kid and HATED by other black kids left a deep mark on my soul and my skin to the point I hated my own black skin. I was so insecure with myself that I would act out to fit in with the wrong crowd. I was acting out because I needed attention and acceptance from my peers.

Being a little black kid and having to eat lunch by yourself and be okay that your family was your only friends… hurt me… hurt me bad. Even these days I don't know how to be "black", because I am Bertrand Harmen Ngampa, I am not just "black". I went so far to fit in and to be accepted that I made some chooses that led me to be kicked out of college.

I fell into depression, anger, suicidal thoughts, and blamed everyone but myself. On the inside I was dying because no one knew my pain of constantly being an outcast. Everywhere I went I felt like I couldn't fit in. It was as if I was designed to fit out and I couldn't handle all that responsibility but on the outside I forcing myself to smile and act as if I had it all together.

Joining the military gave me a place I could connect with and have that feeling of belonging and connection. I was not by myself anymore. I was part of a greater mission than just waking up, going to school, and then dying.

The Army taught me to build my mind, train my body, connected me back to my soul, and know my money. More importantly, God sent people into my life to help me, but in the end, I had to reap what I had sowed into my life. I overcame some of it but to be completely transparent I am still overcoming many demons and issues from childhood.

In closing, everything I have written in this book has helped or is helping me now to get results so I may reach my next level! I pray that this book gives you the words, the clarity, the insight, the guidance and it becomes your personal manual to get results.

And to you that don't fit in anywhere. Add me on Facebook.

Remember the ones that are different change the world.

Follow Me Now: Facebook: Bertrand Ngampa | Instagram: bngampa

Theme I Mind

"Mind over matter." If you played sports before, then you have probably heard this saying before. "Your body is weak, but your mind is strong." I heard that during my time at Army Basic Training. And it has stuck with me even till today. I could keep posting "fancy" quotes, but, in all, you need to know your results in life starts with your mind.

Your mind is the most powerful tool you have and once you get it thinking in the right direction you will become unstoppable.

"But B, how do I get my mind to think in the right direction for results in my life?"

I am glad you asked, I love explaining this, because it is simple to say but hard to do.

You must discover and write down your "why." Your "why" is your personal statement to your mind telling it your reasons you must get theses results!

Answer these Questions.

Why do you want to reach your next level?

What purpose does maximizing your results in each of your life pillars hold?

- Mind?

- Body?

- Soul?

- Money?

Are you ready to do whatever it takes to get results in your mind?

Your answers to these questions will help you to start thinking more deeply about your "why."

When you have a "why" you understand the reason you are going to go home and cook instead of going thru an unhealthy fast food drive thru. When you have a "why" you understand the reason you are going to invest in drink Kangen water or getting a total house alkaline system. When you have a "why" you understand the reason you are dropping friends, family, and co-workers who add no value to your life. When you have a "why" you understand the reason you are going to wake up early or stay up late building your business. When you have a "why" you understand the reason you are going to accept your life at the present moment, however you know you must and will do whatever it takes to maximize your results in your life. When you have a "why" you set your mind to start flowing in the right direction for you to achieve the next level in your life.

Like I said above your "why" is your personal statement to your mind telling it your reasons you must get these results.

Priming Your Mind For Results

Results start by seeing them in your mind. You must transfer what you see in your mind into words, those words into phrases, and those phrases into sentences. Ultimately known as your personal affirmations.

 Before you create your personal affirmations, you must start to starve your "want" list and feed your "have" and "must" list.

How many times have you told yourself you want to do X, Y, Z, A, B, C, 1, 2, 3, 99, and 100, but you never did anything on that "want" list. (I'm so guilty of this all the time!!!!)

When you "want" to do anything you will not do it because the motivation and feelings behind a "want" will die out before you accomplish it. Your "want" list changes quicker than your emotions.

Who else beside me is guilty of telling themselves, "After work I will do X, Y, Z, A, B, C, 1, 2, 3, 99, and 100." But after work comes and you have no energy and that feeling of "want" leaves you. Because your bed is calling your name, you're scrolling endlessly on social media to save your life, and or you promise yourself tomorrow it will get done and then tomorrow never comes, because tomorrow is not promised to you.

So you cannot promise to put off a goal in a future that is not promised to you. (Too deep?) Your want list tells your mind that these items are not important and to not focus on it.

Start feeding your "have" mentality. When you have to do something, you will do it. Going to work, paying rent, paying bills, drinking water, eating food, going to the bathroom, are the basic haves of life. Your have list tells your mind these are top priorities.

Want List	Have List
Go to the movies	Pay Rent by the 1st of each month
Clean my room	Go to work by 8am Monday thru Friday
Call my brother	Email my boss by 5 pm today

Want list: Depending on your energy level and emotions it will probably not get done and push off till tomorrow and probably never get done.

Have list: Whether you have energy or not, you will do these items today or in the next couple days.

Must list: Doesn't matter even if Jesus is coming back today! It is done! (pun intended)

You should now understand to start building a **have and must** list only, so your mind can be active in helping you accomplish these goals. Every time you accomplish your list, you will reach another level in one of your life pillars.

(P.S life pillars are your mind, body, soul, and money)

Your Words, U.S Army, and You

When I talk about affirmations 99.99% of people don't believe their words matter or influence their life at all. Your words matter so much. Your words can change your life. Affirmations are words, phrases, and sentences you say to build your life's pillars. Examples of Affirmations

I am beautiful.

I am brilliant.

I am worthy.

I am conscious of who I am.

I attract the right mentors who graciously share their knowledge and wisdom with me.

Every day in every way I am improving my life pillars for my health.

> *1 Thessalonians 5:11*
>
> *Therefore encourage one another and build one another up, just as you are doing.*

Every morning at Army basic training (boot camp) we would yell the Solider Creed before Breakfast. Look at the Soldier Creed and let me know what you notice.

Soldier Creed

I am an American Soldier.

I am a warrior and a member of a team.

I serve the people of the United States, and live the Army Values.

I will always place the mission first.

I will never accept defeat.

I will never quit.

I will never leave a fallen comrade.

I am disciplined, physically and mentally tough, trained and proficient in my warrior tasks and drills.

I always maintain my arms, my equipment and myself.

I am an expert and I am a professional.

I stand ready to deploy, engage, and destroy, the enemies of the United States of America in close combat.

I am a guardian of freedom and the American way of life.

I am an American Soldier.

 The Soldier's Creed are a list of affirmations that we spoke from a point of already being what we say. If the greatest military in the world have their own affirmations, why don't you have your own personal affirmations?

Did you know the most sought after book in the world is full of affirmations too? Do you know the book? Yes, you guessed it: The Holy Bible. It is full of affirmations. Just open it up and you will read affirmations like these listed below and throughout this manual.

Jeremiah 29:11

11 For I know the plans I have for you," declares the LORD, "plans to prosper you and not to harm you, plans to give you hope and a future.

Psalm 23

A psalm of David

1 The LORD is my shepherd, I lack nothing.

2He makes me lie down in green pastures, he leads me beside quiet waters,

3 he refreshes my soul. He guides me along the right paths for his name's sake.

4 Even though I walk through the darkest valley, I will fear no evil, for you are with me; your rod and your staff, they comfort me.

5 You prepare a table before me in the presence of my enemies. You anoint my head with oil; my cup overflows.

6Surely your goodness and love will follow me all the days of my life, and I will dwell in the house of the LORD forever.

Philippians 4:13

13 **I can do all this through Christ** who gives me strength.

Isaiah 41:10

10 So do not fear, for I am with you; do not be dismayed, for I am your God. I will strengthen you and help you; I will uphold you with my righteous right hand.

Isaiah 40:31

31 but those who hope in the LORD will renew their strength. They will soar on wings like eagles; they will run and not grow weary, they will walk and not be faint.

Philippians 4:6

6 Do not be anxious about anything, but in every situation, by prayer and petition, with thanksgiving, present your requests to God.

Remember, in the beginning was the Word, and the Word was with God. God spoke the world into existence. Execution followed God's words and the world was made. If we have been given the same power as God, why have you not started to speak your results into your life? {WDS}

(Enough Bible Study lesson, let us move on.)

I created a simple creed also called a list of affirmations you can say every day to start your journey into becoming a result taker.

Result Taker Creed

I am a Result Taker.

I am committed to maximizing my results in my life pillars to reach my next level in life.

I am building my mind.

I am training my body.

I am connecting with my spirit.

I know my money.

I am empowering all those around me to take results from life.

I am taking pride in my country and my countrymen.

I am selfish with my health and taking care of me, so I may take care of those around me.

I am a Result Taker."

{Results Be}, ON ME!

As I close the mind section I want to leave you with this.

Results are NOT given. They are TAKEN!

-Bertrand Ngampa

<u>Recap Time & Execution Plan:</u>

Step 1: Discover and Write down your "WHY?".

Step 2: Build and Write down Have and Must " list"

Step 3: Build and Write down your personal affirmations.

Step 4: Build Time within each day to see and say your "why", "goals", and personal affirmations, and Result Taker Creed every day.

Step 5: Become a Result Taker!

Theme II Body

When I worked in a commercial gym I would have a standard script to follow and ask clients like you on how we can help you change your body.

"Standard script"

"Hello Madam/ Sir,"

(small talk)

"So why do you want to achieve X,Y,Z, 1,2,3 and 99, and 100 for your body?"

(fuel to help me close the sale later)

"Well, perfect. We can help you do that by you coming to work out with us 3-4 times a week. Does this price fit your budget?"

(Usually we shoot high, you say no that is too much and boom the sale starts!)

"Oh no!"

"Well, let's build you a plan that does."

"Standard Script Over"

…. (Snap back Result Taker)

But you get my point. I'm going to flip the script about how you can get real results for your body. P.S. The crazy part about this simple process is that it has been around since the beginning of time.

Before I share this with you, let me ask you, *what are the top 3 survival needs for your body if you were stuck on an island?*

1.

2.

3.

Look how smart you are.

1. Air
2. Water
3. People
4. Food   (There's 4! .. "but Coach B you only ask for 3…?)

Yes! I know (insert your name here), but the same top 3 survival needs for the body are the same top 3 that will help you maximize your results to reach your next level in your body. Let us breath deeper as we dive into #1. (pun intended)

Air Is KING.

You could have all the water, people, food, money, and anything you want but without air you will NEVER enjoy it.

You can only hold your breath for so long until you die. So, Air is #1 and I'm going to guess you agree --_* ← (winky face.) Now you understand why air is important but how you use your air also known as breathing is important too.

Breathing Through Your Belly

By breathing correctly you will start getting results in your body. Now this is another simple process. All you must do is switch your chest breathing to belly breathing, also known as diaphragmed breathing, deep breathing, and deep diaphragmatic breathing. (I call it belly breathing- so much easier! Don't you agree?)

Simple 7 Steps to Belly Breathing

Try this right now and let me know how it goes!

Step 1: Put your palm on your belly button.

Step 2: Breathe all the air in your nose you can, while allowing that air to fill your belly. (Side note: Your belly should expand, but your chest should not move)

Step 3: Hold for 1 second.

Step 4: Breathe all the air out thru mouth, while allowing your belly to deflate.

Step 5: Hold for 1 second.

Step 6: Repeat step 2 through 4.

Step 7: Do it for 1 minute, while repeating step 2 through 4. (Side note: Work up to 5 minutes)

You can do this standing, sitting, walking, and thru out your day.

Make these a habit and switch from chest to belly breathing and watch your results come in!

Just by spending 5 minutes when you wake up belly breathing, may cause you to experience some if not all benefits listed below and much more.

Key Benefits of Belly Breathing

- Oxidized blood (Increase Alkalinity)
- Increase Natural Energy
- Reduce Stress
- Increase Awareness
- Increase Focus
- Increase Clarity
- Natural High (FREE)
- Deeper Sleep (My favorite!!!)
- Deeper Connection to Yourself

I love sleeping and with my hectic schedule I need all the energy I can get. Being able to improve my sleep and energy just by switching how I was breathing was huge for me.

How easy was that and look at those benefits. Which one would you like to have?

What if you could have all these benefits above plus more just by drinking more water. Would you start drinking water?

Why We LOVE Water (And You Should Too!)

Your body is made up of 70% water and everything within your body are made up largely of water as well. According to science..

Did you know your Brain is made up of about 70 %?

Did you know your Blood is made up of about 80 %?

Did you know your Skin is made up of about 75 %?

Did you know your Liver is made up of about 68 %?

Did you know your Kidney is made up of about 80 %?

Did you know your Muscles is made up of about 60 %?

Did you know your Bones made up of about 22 %?

Did you know your Lungs is made up of about 79 %?

Did you know your Heart is made up of about 79 %?

From all this you can see why water is a 2nd HUGE step for maximizing your results in your body! Your intake of water will change your body. When you are properly hydrated, you will start to empower your body to reach its own next level.

Benefits of Proper Hydration {WD&S}

- Zero Calories
- Increases Energy levels
- Decrease Belly Fat
- Decreases your Fatigue levels
- Improves Skin's Feel, Look, and Touch
- Increase Immune System
- Flushes out Toxins
- Promotes Weight Loss within the body
- Natural Decreases appetite & Cravings
- Increases metabolism
- … and so much MORE!!!!

Super Hydration Routine

Upon waking up, do your 5 minutes of belly breathing routine and right after, I want you to drink 2 cups of warm water. Yes! I said WARM water. Try it before you knock it! Work your way up to drinking 5 to 8 cups of warm water.

(It is more beneficial for your body to drink warm water when you wake up.)

I am a firm believer in the power of water, but did you know the kind of water you drink matters too. Not all waters are equal. You have tap water, bottled water, and alkaline bottled water, and my personal favorite alkalized water.

Tap Water

Unless you live in Flint, Michigan, then your tap water looks safe to drink. However, your tap water is not as healthy as you may believe and most people don't drink their tap unless they boil it first.

Your tap water is treated with a host of chemicals and there are certain limits on the level of contaminants that are allowed in your water.

Why are there limits on the level of contaminants, how about no contaminants?

Keep reading if you Agree?

Bottled Water

Everyone points to bottle water as being the healthier alternative to sugar laden juices, soda, and or tap water. But what if I told you bottled water is just tap water at a cost. Read your bottled water label if it says "Municipal sources"... they got you twice.

Meaning you paid your water bill and they took your same tap water from your sink and bottled it up and sold it to you for pure profit! If anything, tap water is healthier because it has more regulation on it than bottled water.

Alkaline Bottled Water

Right now there is a huge push and everyone around me is going for alkaline bottled water. Which I am all about improving your body but let me share some insight with you.

Alkaline bottle water is a chemical change meaning they had to add chemicals to the water to increase the alkalinity of the water. If you drink this, you may experience some of the dangers over time associated with alkaline water.

Alkalized Water

Alkalized water means you shock the water with electricity. No added chemicals, however you get all the benefits.

In my home right now, I have a machine from Enagic called a SD 501 that makes Kangen water and helps to remove contaminants*, chlorine*, lead*, and alkalizes my water. (*Known to get rid of 90% of contaminants, chlorine, and lead*)

You may experience some if not all of these benefits when you start drinking Alkalized water:

- Deeper Sleep
- Less Pains and Aches
- Quicker Recovery Time
- Strengthens the body's immune system
- Decrease Free-radicals in the body
- Faster & Better Hydration
- Your pet will love it

- Your kids will love it
- Your skin will glow
- Your nails will grow faster
- Your hair will be soft and full
- May help with asthma*
- May help with allergies*

What if you could have all these benefits plus more just by drinking more alkalized water? Would you start drinking more alkalized water today?

(P.S. If you any questions and or care about your families' body and/or your own body and you want to experience the benefit of alkalized water listed above everyday within your own home send me a message right now.)

How To Make Your Plain Water Enjoyable To Drink

I understand after you drink 1 or 2 gallons of water it is hard to keep drinking water. It has no taste and you want some flavor. Well here is a few ways you can make your water enjoyable to drink.

- **Add Lemons or Limes To Your Water**
  - Adding lemons and limes turns your water into lemonade and limeade but absolute in no situation should you add sugar!!!
  - Lemons and Limes are alkaline when they enter the body which causes many benefits to your body.
- **Add Fruits & Veggies To Your Water**
  - Adding squeezed natural fruit juices to your water is great.
  - Adding cut up fruits to your water and the whole fruit into the water too.
    - Oranges, Strawberries, Cucumbers, and blueberries just some ideas.
- **Add Herbs To Your Water**
  - Passionfruit, Mint, Basil.. etc
- **Make a tea (None caffeinate & No sugar)**
  - Green tea
  - Black tea
  - DON'T ADD SUGAR

<u>We Talking About People… People… Not Food… But People</u>

<u>-Allen Inversion Bertrand Ngampa</u>

People always look at me and are baffled when I state the 3rd item you need to survive is (drum roll please) PEOPLE!

Not food! What you mean!? You lying! HOW! WHAAAAAT!

-People in disbelief

Yes, not food. If you were on an island you would need air, clean water, and people to survive. But Bertrand, I don't live on an island I live in the suburbs. Yes, I understand, but understand it is not just people; it is the connection with people.

We are meant to be connected with other people. That is why solitary confinement is the worst punish for you.

Who are you connected with daily, weekly, monthly, and yearly!?

People you are connected with affect your life more than you know!

!!!!!!!! STORY TIME !!!!!!!!

When I was a personal trainer. I told this lady she may have to drop her friends and their opinions.

Right away, her so-called friends told her "why do you want to lose weight? Didn't you already try that? Come on girl! You know you not going to do that! Stop Girl Byeee!" Damn, that is not what I call friends but I empowered and closed her to make the decision to work with me.

Even her boyfriend told me, "She will not last. She will quit soon."

When I say that everyone doubted her, they did not encourage her, and were all waiting for her to fail. I MEAN it. I had to step up and empower her with affirmations and help her to see that everyone around her was not for her.

At first, she was constant and it was going good but then her so-called friends word's got into her ears and told her "come out with us", "you changed", "you are not fun anymore".

So, she went out with them. But my affirmations I sowed in her must of have fully grown while she was out because she texted me as she was out.

"I can't keep living like this! Fuck everyone that doesn't believe in me. I want this and I need your help. I'm sorry for being missing will you help me please?"

The next day we met at the gym and every day after we would work out together. She would secretly workout twice a day and even her mind shifted from negative to more positive.

Her boyfriend told me. "the things that used to make her upset don't and she is just more happy and free." She told me she would use affirmations at work when it got stressful to help her to calm down.

She even started to make friends with new more positive friends at the gym and her actions encouraged many others to look at their own health. Her results would blow your mind away. It blew my mind away when I saw it. But I can not take all the credit because she did all the work and now she has her results plus she is helping others to reach their next level.

!!!!!! END OF STORY !!!!!

Your so called friend can't have you do the "impossible" because it leaves them no excuse to why they can't accomplish it either.

Connect with individuals that will push, inspire, and empower you to take results from life.

****Side Bar Major Key: People that believe you and them are on the same level pray for your downfall when you set a goal because WHEN you accomplish that goal they can't hide behind their excuses anymore. Side Bar Major Key Over*****

I hope you see the real meaning behind theses short story and amazing artistic picture above that people you connect with can affect your life pillars in tremendous ways. When you allow connections to grow with people you are allowing them to speak into your life.

Whether you agree or disagree with what they say, their words may leave a scar on your life. All of us have a human desire of wanting to be connected and understood.

It is a human desire that is more powerful than any food or water.

You can survive months without food but you can only survive 3 days without fresh water, and only minutes without air. It makes sense now why people (connections) is Step 3.

> *Proverbs 13:20 Walk with wise men, and thou shalt be wise; But the companion of fools suffers harm.*

Recap Time & Execution Plan

Questions to Ask yourself about Friends. (Growth comes with Awareness)

Why are your friend's friends with you?

Do you add value or take value from their life?

Do they add value or take value from your life?

Do you motivate, empower, and push your friends to reach their next level?

Do you speak life or death into your friend's life pillars?

Why am I friends with him or her?

Does he or she add value or take value from my life?

Do my current friends motivate, empower, and or push me to reach my next level?

What do I look for in a friend?

Do your friends speak life or death into your life pillars?

Are you and your friends on the same level? Are they above or below you? Are they helping you up or dragging you down?

List your top 3 friends. Next to their name write why you are friends.

1.
2.
3.

Do you need a new group of friends?

Do you need to delete any friends from your life?

Are you strong enough to walk away from current friend/ friends and make seek friends?

Proverbs 18: 21

"Life and death are held in the power of the tongue, those who love to talk will have to eat their own words.

Theme III Soul

I am about to get really hippie, hooky, spiritually, and whatever else you want to call it!

We are going to dive deep into your SOUL pillar.

Feed the soul, and you will never be hungry.

Our Soul's long for connections. In the previous chapter I told you how the people you are related to effect your body. The same concept holds true for your soul.

Now the Soul pillar is a little deeper connection because this is your spouse and or other significant connections. When your spouse is trying to reach their next level, you should empower and encourage them with your words and actions to do so.

Many times the problem with this comes when women are the "bread winner" and men have to motivate, empower, and push their wife to reach their next level. Most times I see men get jealous and start to bring their wife down and belittle her from reaching their next level.

> *I should have said this in the beginning, but never allow societies' norm or rules keep you from reaching your next level.*
>
> *-Bertrand Ngampa #BFiT*

Before I go on, let me talk about the Soul pillar in a more personal selfish type of way. Within all of us we have a conscious and subconscious mind. Not to get too deep on you but I'll breakdown both conscious and subconscious.

Conscious mind: Can be turned on and off. It can be used to program your subconscious mind.

Subconscious mind: It cannot be turned off. It is on 24/7. You program it to attract what you want out of life.

Your conscious mind is the captain of the ship and the subconscious mind is the ship. The Ship doesn't decide on whether the captain's orders are good or bad, it does whatever the captain says to do. So, if the captain is leading it to the rocks (also known as danger) then it will go towards the rocks without questions.

Therefore affirmations are important. They sow seeds in your subconscious mind and at the right or wrong time they grow and sprout into action in your life.

Affirmations are good and bad.

For example, when you wake up you affirm your day with.

"Today is a great day!"

or

"Today is going to suck!"

You choose what today will be like for you.

Matthew 21:22 NIV

If you believe, you will receive whatever you ask for in prayer."

How To Feed Your Soul

During my time at Integrative Institute of Nutrition (IIN) I learned there are two types of food. Primary and secondary food.

Primary food: Health Relationship, Spiritually practice, Passionate work, and Exercise

Secondary Food: Food on your plate that you physically eat.

It don't matter how many green juices you drink or super foods you eat if you have not taken care of your primary food you will "never" be truly healthy.

-IIN

You and I can both agree we know many people that go to gym everyday but they are full of stress, have no mindset, and overall their life pillars are not in place.

"You could go to the gym every day and still not be healthy."

- *Bertrand Ngampa #BFiT*

Examples of Primary Food

Health Relationships: Have you ever been with a special someone that the conversation is sooo good you forget about everything else in life and your only focus is the person before you? Think back on the time of your 1st date with your spouse or significant other. Remember that feeling you got when that person you secretly had a crush on in grade school would talks to you?

(P.S A healthy relationship is full of acceptance for who you are at that moment. No judgment but you are honestly held accountability.)

Spiritual Practice: Have you ever been at your place of worship or the house of your God, Gods, and or Goddesses and you are on a "spiritually high" that you feel as if you have been elevated and at that moment everything else fades away?

(A church is not the only place to find God. I found God 2000ft in the sky before I jumped out a C-17. Airborne!)

Passionate Work: Have you ever been doing an action that aligns with your views to the "T" that you would rather see the action to completion before taking a break.

(Example for the example: Mission trip, talking with "homeless" people, and part-time hustle. Till this day I remember going on a mission trip to North Carolina and I met this little girl named Hope. Even though she had "nothing" she was the happiest little girl in the world. My youth group and I didn't even take a break the whole time and always worked through lunch.)

Exercise: After a hard workout that leaves you exhausted and pushed beyond your limits. You start to think about your life in a deeper way. Nothing matters beside laying there and just trying to survive.

(That is what Day 00 is like for all my training clients. My training causes them to dig deep and push themselves pass their excuses and their "I can't do anymore" mindset.)

From all these examples, I hope you could relate or had similar situations in your life.

> *Results in your Soul pillar start with your Primary food, not your Secondary food.*
>
> *-Bertrand Ngampa #BFiT*

Let's touch on Secondary food. Remember Secondary food being food on your plate.

1. **Listen To Your Body**

i. So, important, we have lost touch with our bodies. Your body will tell if you eat something that it agrees or disagree with.

ii. Example: Animal dairy makes many people get upset stomach, bloating, and acne after eating it. They know it and continue to eat it instead of finding an alternative or eliminating it from their life.

2. **Eat Real Food**

i. Limit processed and package food. Eat food that is normally found in natural or close to it. Use your stove top more and microwave less. Follow my Less and More list to get maximize result in your secondary food.

3. **Eat For Your Gut.**

i. Take care of the inside of your body and give it all it needs to function and you will reap the benefits on the outside of your body.

Less Of This	*More Of This*
Less process food	More REAL naturally food
Less fried food	More baked/ broiled food
Less processed meat	More "real" meat
Less dining out	More "dining in" your house
Less drinking alcohol & juice	More Kangen water & filtered water
Less candy	More fruits & vegetables
Less white flour	More whole wheat flour
Less stress	More gratitude

Recap Time & Execution Plan

Secondary food is simple.

Overall the biggest take away: Primary food is more important than the secondary food!

Feed your Soul 1st! You can't feed your Soul with secondary food and expect to reach your next level.

- *Bertrand Ngampa*

Theme IIII Money

Money is the root of all evil.

If you believe that above statement. You may be poor (mindset), broke (state of having no money), always asking others for money, and or never have enough money...

"It is okay to be broke, but never say you are poor again!"

> *-Coach B*

Money nowadays is just a piece of paper with a number attached to it. Back in the day money used to be gold, silver, sheep, ox, seashells, silk, and whatever else was deemed valuable.

Money is not good or evil, it is a paper with a number attached to it.

I love making money and knowing my money. My favorite day is payday, because I can take my money and go do whatever my money allows me to do.

Nowadays there is two ways to make money. Work a traditional job or Own your own business.

Let's talk about the traditional route and how we can maximize your results to get more money out of your job.

OWNER

Corporate Goons

Middle Management

YOU

Let pretend you are at the bottom of the barrel and you make livable money. Nothing crazy but you can pay your rent and almost always pay all your bills. In a traditional job if you want to make more money, you need to increase your value to the company.

(Side note - Excuse me before we go any further lets both agree no matter what you do, you will never be the owner of this company because it is not your company. Okay? Okay!)

Ways To Increase Your Value To Your Company

- Get a degree
- Specialize in a certain area to help the company
- Be on time
- Work harder than everyone else

Let me stop there because at the end of the day if you want to make more money at your traditional job right now it comes down to 2 simple things.

1. **Work more hours (Hourly)**
    i. If you are an hourly employee working more hours and diving into overtime (time and half) will certainly show on your next paycheck.
2. **Move up within your company (Salary)**
    i. Getting a promotion usually comes with a raise in pay.
3. **If you are in commission (Sales)**
    i. Make more sales!

Yes! You must work hard, out work your peers, be on time, but to get those RESULTS that lead you to the money you want from your job you must either work more hours and or move up within the company.

Too easy?

Too Easy!

Let's Breakdown Owning Your Own Business!

I always tell my clients to find a part time business or side hustle they can do on top of their job.

Before I get back to owning your own business, I know many of my clients have always told me how they hate their job and or they are scared for the future a.k.a retirement. Yet, when I tell them about owning their own business they can't fathom it.

They always use excuses like, "I'm too old, that cost too much, I don't have time, and whatever excuse they can think of."

It is so easy to start a business, answer theses 2 questions.

What are your passions and interest?

Out of everything you like to do, which one can you start to make money from?

Now right now I know what you are thinking. "No one will pay me for (insert your passions and interest)." I tell everyone this, if people make a livable wage to post videos of themselves having sex online you can get paid to (insert your passions and interest here).

Another example, kids, and I'm talking 18 years old and younger make six figures plus from making funny videos online. Another example, air is 25 cents at the gas station and even a whole 4 quarters at some places!

What does that mean????? That means even air which is free has a price!

Did you know to have a baby at the hospital they will charge you money?

That means you reading this right now, you, had a price tag to be born.

I say allllll that to say! No matter what your passion or interest are you can monetize it!

The point I hope to drive into your mind is that no matter what your passion or interest are there is room for you to turn it into a business or a side hustle.

!!!!!!!!!!!!! Story Time Again!!!!!!!!!!!!!!!!!!

How I missed out on **$4000+** from not starting my own business

Before I started my own personal training business, I was full of fear and excuses. I am so passionate about health and fitness that I used to train and give out my knowledge for free.

It was not until a lady I gave free advice to and well over $4000+ worth of value for free. I wrote her a workout program, detailed hourly meal plan, affirmations, and even access to me whenever she needed it. Did I tell you I charged her $0 dollars?

She took everything I gave her and did not use one thing!

People don't value free.

!!!!!!!!!!!!!! END OF STORY!!!!!!!!!!!!!!

However, I did pre-sell her on the idea that she needed a personal trainer. So, when she went to a gym and invested $750 a month for a "Master Trainer" that offered her just a workout plan. And that was a 6-month plan she signed up for too.

"Master" Gym Trainer Workout Plan (Value $750)	Bertrand Ngampa Workout plan (Valued $1000) Meal plan ($500) Affirmations ($500) Access to me (Total Value $5000)
Investment: $750	Investment: $0

People don't value free.

This Master Trainer and I on paper are both the same. The difference between him and I are our personality, knowledge, and our perfect "ideal" customer. Oh, I forget 1 thing, he made the decision to start his own personal training business and threw out his fear and excuses. Even after I learned about the whole above situation I still made many excuses like the ones below.

I don't have the experience to run a personal training.

What if I fail?

Why would anyone come work with me, when there are many other successful trainers in my area?

What if no one wants to buy?

What if my prices are too high?

I am only 21 years old, who is going to take me serious?

I don't have enough money for a website, business cards, and other fitness tools needed.

The list went on for about 6-months .. until I decided to start my business without any website, business cards, and other fitness tools. I got a certification and worked with what I had.

Again, I say all that, so you would throw out your excuses and start your business or side hustle now! It doesn't need to be perfect you must start it and focus on what you have and make that work! Remember nothing is perfect and if you must wait till it is perfect you will never start.

Side note: Sometimes when you are reaching your next level it doesn't look pretty and or perfect.

Simply 2 things you must do that will result as making more money at your job right now

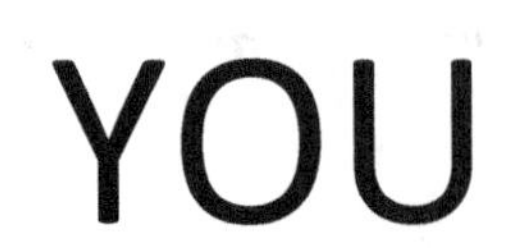

Remember we can both agree you will never own this company because it is not your company!

Only 2 ways that will result in more money for you at your pyramid scheme. I mean job. (lol moment)

1. **Work more hours**
    i. If you are an hourly employee working more hours and diving into overtime (time and ½) will certainly show on your next paycheck.
2. **Move up within your company**
    i. Getting a promotion usually comes with a raise in pay. (Most time it is more work and not enough pay)

How To Start Your Own Business And Or Side Hustle

Answer these questions

What are your top 10 passions and interest?

1.
2.
3.
4.
5.
6.
7.
8.
9.
10.

Out of all your passion and interest, circle which one can you start to make money from now!

Major Hint Key:

Think of a problem in your community. Solve that problem in your community.

How can your passion or interest solve a problem in your community?

Community	Passion & Interest

| "The Problem" | Side Hustle | | "The Solution" |
| | Business | | |

Where your community's problem meets your passion & interest...
your business & side hustle is born!

-Coach B

People don't value free.

Example:

Problem in my community are obesity and high blood pressure.

I partnered with the #1 supplement company in America that target high blood pressure naturally and I offer personal training to people that want to lose weight. Don't forget to charge for your services or product.

(If you are overweight visit www.coachbn.com . If you have high blood pressure or know anyone with high blood pressure that would like to naturally reverse it give them my website www.coachbn.com)

People don't value free.

We could end this book here, because I have shared with you a lot of actionable and valuable information. Let me share some more value with you. This book will not help you with reaching your next level if you just read it and don't take action on it!

What I am about to share with you next helped me to take responsibility of my lack of money from it being evil to it being my own fault.

To know your money means you must know all aspects and not only in your mind but on paper too!

Know Your Money

And the easiest way to do that is by writing down all and I mean ALL your monthly budget, monthly income avenues, your payoff list, and future income avenues.

MONTHLY BUDGET

RENT	1,500
CELL PHONE	100
GAS	100
ELECTRIC	100
WATER	100
FOOD	100
INTERNET	150
CAR PAYMENT	225
TOTAL COST	2,150

Have you written down your monthly number?

Most of you know your budget in your mind but have not written it on paper. People lie, but numbers don't. Declutter your mind by writing your budgets down. If you want the result of more money you MUST write down your monthly budget. Do you know how much you must make to just breakeven every month?

MONTHLY INCOME AVENUES

JOB 1	$2,000 ($500 weekly)
JOB 2	$1,000 ($250 weekly)
SIDE HUSTLE	$600 ($150 weekly)
TOTAL INCOME	$3,600
TOTAL POCKET	$1450

JOHN DOE FUTURE MONTHLY INCOME AVENUES	
JOB 1	$2,000 ($500 weekly)
JOB 2	$1,000 ($250 weekly)
SIDE HUSTLE	$2000 ($500 weekly)
TOTAL INCOME	$5,000
TOTAL POCKET	$2,850

How much more money do you want to make?

How can you know how much more money you must make if you don't know how much you make every month.

 Logically thinking you should not go out and spend more than your weekly income or put myself in a situation where you cannot at least breakeven each month.

The best way to result in more money in your pocket would be to look at all your income avenues and decide where you can increase your income avenues in.

For example, if John Doe increased his side hustle from $600 a month to $2000 a month, he will add $1400 a month to his total pocket.

If you could add any extra $1400 into your income to spend, save, invest, and or do whatever. Would buying "healthy" food be expensive?

Would "Money" still be evil?

How can you add an extra $100, $500, $1400 to your pocket?

PAYOFF LIST	
CREDIT CARD	2500
CAR	25,000
KANGEN MACHINE	4,950
TOTAL NETWORTH	-32,450

Payoff List is my favorite one of all. Because people think you need to be a millionaire to live a lavish life but that is far from the truth. All you must do is payoff your debt and gain a positive income flow.

If you were debt-free and any money you made went right into increasing your total positive income flow how much more could you maximize your other life pillars if you were not always concern on your money pillar?

Use these charts to fill in your monthly budget, income avenues, payoff list and be 100% honest with yourself.

Major Hidden Keys

You would be surprised how many times people tell me, "I don't know how much I spend each month and I don't want to know!" People just like you fear knowing their numbers. Stop being fearful, ones you learn your number you can grow that number!

Monthly budget: Put all essentials items on this budgets 1st. Then add all and every item that takes even .01 cent out of your account.

YOUR MONTHLY BUDGET	
RENT	
CELL PHONE	
TOTAL COST	

Income Avenues: Any jobs you hold that give you an amount of income add it. Any business and or side hustle legal or illegal add it too. (Don't show the IRS)

Future income avenues: Where can you make more money within your avenues?

MONTHLY INCOME AVENUES			
JOB 1	$	($	weekly)
JOB 2	$	($	weekly)
SIDE HUSTLE	$	($	weekly)
TOTAL INCOME		$	
TOTAL POCKET		$	

JOHN DOE FUTURE MONTHLY INCOME AVENUES			
JOB 1	$	($	weekly)
JOB 2	$	($	weekly)
SIDE HUSTLE	$	($	weekly)
TOTAL INCOME		$	
TOTAL POCKET		$	

Payoff List: Write down all the areas you owe any money, no matter how small or big.

YOUR PAYOFF LIST

*Money is needed to get results and reach your next level. Please understand to make more money means you **MUST** give more value to your market place.*

P.S Owning your own business is not for everyone and I understand that completely. But **living paycheck to paycheck** is not ideal either. You must get uncomfortable and learn some new skills that will result in more money.

If you work a tradition job and are completely happy at it. I am happy for you and now you know the simple 2 steps in making more money at your job right now!

Recap Time & Execution Plan

To close the money theme, let me start by again stating, money is not evil or the root of all evil. Money is now just a piece of paper with a number attached to it. If you want to reach the next level and maximize your money pillar at your traditional job you must do 2 things;

1. **Work more hours**
2. **Move up within the company**

(Side note: We can agree a 3rd time you can never own the company because it is not your company!)

You may not of known how to start your business or side hustle in the beginning however list 10 passion and interest and decide what you can start making money from now..

Even if you don't do anything else. KNOW YOUR MONEY in and out! Keep track of how much goes in and out. How much extra money you must spend, save, and or INVEST.

Result Taker

PHEW! Dry up the tears and just breath, it will be okay. I'm not going to overwhelm you with more actionable information. But I want to thank you for taking the time and reading your book. I am proud of you for investing in your own life, life pillars, and those around you. The results you get from this book whether they are small or completely 180-degree life changing it will be felt and noticed by those around you.

Here is my last task for you.

1. **Build Your Mind**
2. **Train Your Body**
3. **Connect With Your Soul**
4. **Know Your Money**

Ask and it will be given to you; seek and you will find; knock and the door will be opened to you

Matthew 7:7

This book is your manual to helping you maximize & dominate your results in your life, so you may reach your next level. If you constantly make those decisions to reach your next level, you will certainly reach your next level. Keep this manual close and open it often. Take a week and work on executing each Theme. When you are finished do it again and keep reaching new levels!

Most people that heard me speak about this or I share this idea with before I wrote this book always ask me.. so How much is it to work with you?

If you are interested in working with me and becoming a RESULT TAKER, apply here:

www.Coachbn.com

My personal client story I love is a beautiful lady that used to wear make up to cover up what was going on and put on a front. However, as we started working together and she started saying these affirmations and taking action on them.

She started to wear less make-up and her natural beauty started to show and glow thru her. Her self-confident, self-esteem, and self-awareness about herself as a woman went up too.

She told me "I would never or could never go to work without make-up," now that her staff has seen her without make up more frequently they tell her she doesn't need it and that her natural face is more than enough.

She started to reach her next level by saying, believing, and taking action on the affirmations we personally built for her life and life pillars.

We started with her mind which flowed to her spirit and now she wants to start taking care of her body and because of her new confidence. Guess what, she is inspiring her sister and other women around her to increase their awareness too.

After you apply, I will give you a call and explain how to become a RESULT TAKER and if you match my ideal client, I will invite you to work with me. Think about this: you could be working personally with me your Results Coach to change your life forever. Are you my ideal client? Go to the website above and take action!

Thank you for reading this book, I pray for massive RESULTS in your LIFE, LIFE PILLARS, and FOR EVERYONE THAT YOU LOOK AT, SPEAK TO, and THINK OF. May God Keep You & Bless You.

RESULTS BE! ON YOU!